Massaging Women

I0843103

Learn the attitudes and approaches
necessary in the light of #MeToo

Develop a safe, trusted practice and
that reflects the reality of women's lives

by Oliver Chapman

A Quick-Start Guide for Therapists in the Age of #MeToo

MASSAGING WOMEN

CONTENTS

A Quick-Start Guide for Therapists in the Age of #MeToo

MASSAGING WOMEN

A Quick-Start Guide for Therapists in the Age of #MeToo

Introduction

Hi! Welcome to *Massaging Women: A Quick-Start Guide for Therapists in the Age of #MeToo.*

No doubt that, as a qualified and certified massage therapist, you are good at what you do and whether you are in private practice or work in a clinic or elsewhere, you know pretty much how to give a good massage and have probably had some training in ethics to deal with client safety issues and their sense of comfort with you as a touch-based therapist.

How is it, then, that one still often hears, on online messageboards or just through the grapevine, of clients feeling uncomfortable with the attitude of their therapists, of therapists taking liberties with the power dynamic between therapist and client, or simply stories of how some therapists feel uncomfortable with certain types of client behaviour in the massage room?

Further, while any client could complain like this, are not many of these clients women?

This Quick-Start Guide has therefore been written with the female client in mind. While some of what I describe could apply to any client, this Guide has been specifically written for therapists dealing with women clients.

Many of the negative comments received from female clients are related in some way to the therapist's non-conformance to the reality of women's lives due to the therapist's lack of knowledge of what women have to put up with outside the massage room. While this lack of knowledge could once be at least partly justified by either a male therapist being unaware or a female therapist attempting to uphold ethics guidelines written by men, this part-justification can no longer safely continue.

A range of events have taken place in public life regarding the bad behaviour of some famous names in the realm of sexual misconduct and these, together with the resultant reactions to them, have led to a movement summed up by the Twitter hashtag #MeToo.

#MeToo was started by Tarana Burke in 2006, an activist for the rights of women and girls in minority communities. More recently, a sexual misconduct scandal involving Hollywood producer Harvey Weinstein led to actress Alyssa Milano asking other women, on Twitter, to use the hashtag if they had experienced similar things.

An astonishingly huge number of women responded, in such vast numbers that the long-held "a third of women have experienced assault" was proved to be correct and probably an understatement. Since then, #MeToo has continued to evolve and question many of the assumptions people have held about the nature of the society we live in and the reality of life most women have to lead.

What made #MeToo so different to other movements prior was that, for the first time, men couldn't dismiss it as a faraway issue. Reports of assault or rape have been heard in the news for a long time but for the man in the street, it always seemed to happen to women he didn't know. It was always some Hollywood actress in LA, or supermodel in Milan or some tribeswomen in Africa or women in the Middle East or some other group of women that he would never meet, knew nothing about and that didn't really affect him. Sure, he would read about it in the papers on his morning commute but, other than shaking his head at the state of the world, what else could he do about it?

#MeToo changed all that. Suddenly, his mum, his sister, his aunt, even his grandmother were saying, "Me, too" on Twitter. He found out some creepy guy followed his sister home three days ago. Some loser grabbed his mum's butt in the supermarket yesterday. Another guy yelled sexual

4

remarks at his grandmother when she was walking her dog in the park.

Then, when he stopped off at Starbucks for his morning coffee, the barista who usually serves him said she got assaulted outside a club two days ago. Then, at work, five women in the office also admitted that similar things happened to them. Then there was the waitress at the diner at lunchtime and the girl at the bus stop and on and on and on...

The upshot of all this is that massage therapists need to adjust their behaviour to suit this "new" reality, which, in fact, isn't new for women at all but is now out in the open. It won't do to either be ignorant or feign ignorance.

Ethics are all well and good but exact ethical practices in the massage room must be reviewed in the light of women's lived experiences.

Assuming that every woman you meet is a rape or assault survivor is a good start. However, that, in turn, raises issues of how best to be ethical in one's practice. If we do everything by the book and follow the same rules of ethics of every healthcare professional, such as doctors, nurses and others, then for sure the opportunity for mistakes will be minimized. Nevertheless, we are healers of a different ilk.

Many rape survivors say most of the lasting trauma is not about the penis or the sperm of their rapist or anything physical that happened but the sense of a lack of control over the outcome, the fear and the shame.

A good massage therapist should know that this fear, shame and trauma will translate into muscle tension, seized-up joints, headaches and other psychosomatic phenomena better dealt with via massage than by a bunch of pills prescribed by a doctor. Yet some of these female clients still have to deal with the power differential between therapist and client and put up with sleazy therapists trying to get something sexy via the massage table.

This Quick-Start Guide, then, aims to address these issues by suggesting a way to meet the needs of these female clients.

CHAPTER ONE

Review Your Knowledge

As a qualified therapist, you probably know much about musculature and the role skeletal muscle plays on the human body. Further, you may also have some basic knowledge of hormones, lactic acid build-up and the processes of cell excretion and how impurities are collected by the lymphatic system and removed from the body.

Before embarking on a wholesale marketing of female clients, however, you might do well to brush up on female-exclusive anatomy and physiology. When people hear "female anatomy" they immediately think of sex organs but that's hardly the whole picture and, indeed, knowledge of genitalia is likely to be of limited value to an ethics-bound practice.

More important is the fact that female muscles have a greater number of slow-twitch muscle fibres than men, which means less power but more endurance. Added to their higher pain threshold, you shouldn't be overly fearful of pressing too hard during your massage.

Further, knowledge of hormonal fluctuations during their menstrual cycle will help you to know which body parts are likely to retain water, which ones get swollen and will therefore be more tender and where menstrual pain is likely to render your massage less pleasant in certain body areas. For example, menstrual pain will mean massage of abdominal areas will be more painful, whereas headaches caused by period pain might mean a head massage would be more appreciated. Women who have had Caesarian sections may have muscle tension in the pelvic area, while pregnant women are a whole specialist area.

You would do wisely to examine your existing female clientele and review your knowledge of them, then decide on what physiological knowledge to brush up on based on their requirements. You can always learn more as

6

your clients' needs change, whether that be through attending seminars, webinars, downloading ebooks like this one, visiting conferences or even formal, face-to-face courses of instruction. Start by assessing your existing clients' needs, study what you need to know, then start. Learn as you go and build up from there.

This book is just a Quick-Start Guide to point you in the right direction. There isn't space or time here to go into lots of detail regarding female physiology. I may write another book that is longer and goes into more detail but for now, consider this a heads-up that any serious attempt to serve women clients will probably need you to specialize your knowledge sooner or later and you might as well prepare for it now.

A Quick-Start Guide for Therapists in the Age of #MeToo

CHAPTER TWO

Update Your Attitude

From just the brief overview of #MeToo given in the Introduction, you can plainly see why it is important for therapists to make changes to the way they operate with female clients, so as to enhance their practice and serve those clients better.

How? A lot of the subsequent discussion that has taken place in the light of #MeToo has been about the issue of toxic masculinity. In brief, this is where men have grown up with an attitude that plays out as though women were second-class citizens. This is a large topic and the number of different ways men act out this belief is myriad. So my first recommendation is that you get acquainted with the basics of feminism and especially as it pertains to #MeToo, #TimesUp and toxic masculinity. The discussion is wide-ranging, rigorous and ongoing.

Some of you might groan at the idea of having to study feminism to better understand female clients. Aha! That's exactly the attitude that needs to be eliminated for you to ultimately succeed in the field of female massage.

In a way, you might as well face it. Anyone who plans on massaging women for 20 years, 10 years or even just five and doesn't come out of that experience as a feminist must be a really bad massage therapist. I can't see how you could possibly take female massage seriously, with women taking their clothes off in front of you on a daily basis, the trust that involves, the intimacy engendered, the tales they then feel free to tell, without you coming away from that with at least a "Feminism 101"-level understanding of women's issues. If you have been massaging women for some time already and you have not heard tales of assault, harassment, sexual coercion, attempted rape, stalkers, ex-boyfriends, lousy husbands, bad dates and other "women's talk" stuff, then that basically means YOU'RE DOING IT WRONGLY.

8

So cut to the chase and get up to speed by reading Everyday Feminism online, subscribing to Ms. Magazine, Bitch and Dame and learn everything you can about toxic masculinity. This applies whether you are a male or female therapist, although I tend to imagine female therapists will be more up on this.

Toxic masculinity usually starts at around age 11, although some small boys can exhibit anti-female behaviour earlier than that, pulling girl's hair in class, pinching and poking girls at school – maybe his parents dismissed this with "boys will be boys" or justified his abuse with "if he's mean, that means he likes you" and so much other junk.

Nevertheless, most boys start to experience what feminists call "the patriarchy" at around the age of 11, where continued acceptance of male friendship becomes dependent on feats of sporting skills and physical prowess, ostensibly to impress women in order to obtain sexual favours from them. It also works the other way, with men using women for sex in order to impress the guys. Later, men use achievement at work to impose a glass ceiling on women to exploit women for sex. Policing of open spaces is done with cat-calling, sexist remarks and other behaviours in public.

Now, some background from me. I was physically, mentally and emotionally abused by my father as an infant, so much so that I developed Avoidant Personality Disorder. Later I was teased and bullied at school by boys until I was 16. During all this time, my mother was an absolute rock and tower of strength. Although I was outwardly friendly towards them, I was inwardly fearful of men and boys. I learned early that to share emotions and feelings with men and boys was not safe.

I was rejected by male peers at the age of 11 for reasons I still don't fully understand. This meant I could never return to the company of my former friends. While this was distressing at the time, it also meant that I gained an absolute interest in all things female. This was partly due to the fact that I am straight, plus the high levels of hormones I had in my teenage years; but most of it was from the fear of isolation and loneliness that would result if I did not make friends with women.

A Quick-Start Guide for Therapists in the Age of #MeToo

MASSAGING WOMEN

Typically, if a man gets rejected by a woman, he has the option of returning to lick his wounds with his male friends, who will dismiss her as not worth his time or come up with some other reason in order to make him feel better. I never had that option. It was WOMEN OR NOTHING.

There were no men to go back to – "nothing" was therefore not an option. Either I had to learn how to love women or I would have absolutely no friends at all. I would be completely alone with no emotional connection in my life whatsoever. This prospect engendered in me a dreadful fear of isolation, so that I would spend the remainder of my life surrounded by women and dedicated to serving them as best I could.

This fear, though painful, has served me well as a massage therapist, allowing me to put my female clients' needs first and to feel a sense of unconditional positive regard towards all women, regardless of her background, beliefs or behaviour in the past, present or future.

I have often sensed that this is lacking from male therapists and from some female ones, too. I have struggled for a long time in wondering how I could recreate it in other therapists; therapists who do not share my background, had more social success as teenagers and who have more healthy friendships with men. Basically, they just don't feel enough fear.

How can you treat a woman as a second-class citizen when they're all you've got for human companionship for the duration of your entire life?
If a male therapist takes advantage of a female client, not only does it show that he treats her as though she's "less than" but, to me, it also shows that he feels no fear of losing her. He never thinks, "Oh, my goodness, I can't do that – I'll lose her – she'll tell all her friends, and women will never trust me again – I'll be alone and isolated for the rest of my life!"

He doesn't care whether he loses her or not because he thinks he's got back-up. He's got male friends and people in higher positions who will turn a blind eye and bosses who will sweep it under the carpet. If the client complains, then he'll say she's exaggerating or he'll gaslight her and say what she thought happened actually didn't and use all manner of tired
10

excuses to justify his mistreatment of her. He's not scared at all because he's got the patriarchy behind him.

Can you see now how feminism is important in massage therapy? It's the difference between a successful practice with women and a malpractice lawsuit.

So how can I give you that fear I have felt without you having to experience being punched in the face at two years of age by your own father, thrown in the garbage by "friends" at school or being told you can't be a friend because your epilepsy stops you from being able to catch a ball or kick it in a straight line?

Well, here it is – I want you to be afraid of losing emotional connection and the opportunity to be vulnerable. That's it.

What makes women so wonderful, in my view, is their marvellous emotional competency. I have implicit trust in a woman's emotional understanding of things. Even when logic might disagree with it or point out flaws, her emotional intelligence is on point and, for massage, that's more important.

On a wider scale, though, this also follows through in the #MeToo discussion of what healthy masculinity might look like. Much agreement has been made that men have been taught to suppress their emotions, (except for anger) and to use sex as a way to express emotion. So while women need to feel to have sex, men have to have sex to feel. This is unhealthy for men and damaging to women and the wider society.

Solutions offered include men learning safe ways to express emotions and to not be ashamed of their sexuality. If you are a male therapist, then massaging women is a great way to learn how to do that. While every massage session is about the client and her issues, not you and yours, nevertheless it goes without saying that if we, as therapists, got absolutely nothing out of our jobs except a pay packet and a pat on the back from our boss and the satisfaction of a job well done, then we wouldn't do it for long.

So I want you to be afraid of losing emotional connection and the chance to learn how to be vulnerable from your female clients. Otherwise, you'll always be that guy who "doesn't get it", the guy who's always on the outside looking in, the guy who tried to get a little when he could have got a lot. DON'T BE THAT GUY. If you play your cards right, you'll have more female clients than you'll know what to do with and you'll never need to worry about getting respect from your patriarchal, misogynistic "friends". Hopefully, you'll be able to make new friends with like-minded men and all of us together can make the world a better place, not just for women but for us, too. I'm excited! LET'S DO IT!

Another thing I want you to do is to develop a Rogerian approach to your massage practice. Carl Rogers was an important figure in the counselling movement and the founder of Person-Centred Counselling. While you might not need to follow all his teachings, I feel that all massage therapists should exhibit what Rogers referred to as the Core Conditions -

1/ Unconditional Positive Regard – we maintain as much as possible a positive attitude towards our client. This doesn't mean we have to agree with her decisions and life choices, especially if you feel these are immoral or unethical but that we accept these decisions were taken by her based on her interpretation of the events of her life and on "where she's coming from". We regard her positively without condition based on her intrinsic value as a human being.
2/ Genuineness – we don't put on "airs and graces" or maintain a "professional facade". We relate to the client as a person and talk genuinely and from the heart.
3/ Empathy – we try our best to put our own frame of reference to one side and adopt hers, so that we can feel what she feels, think how she thinks, understand how she understands, so as to create greater connection with her as the client.

These are the Core Conditions needed to create transformations in the counselling room, so if you introduce them into the massage room, with
12

all that physical touch, too, how amazing your massage will be! She will be able to feel these things through your hands – and how awesome that will be for women who have suffered trauma!

Finally, I want you to have what I call a "lover's mentality" towards women, regardless of whether you are a male or female therapist. Although, as professionals, we don't do anything sexy ourselves in the massage room, that doesn't preclude female clients taking matters into their own hands, sometimes literally.

This requires, then, an attitude that, unless proven otherwise, all women are fabulous, amazing creatures of incredible beauty, mystery and passion; that being in their presence is one of the greatest pleasures of this mortal life; that to lead her is to serve her; that whatever you give her, she will always pay back double; that her capacity for pleasure is almost infinite; that her emotional intuition is always trustworthy; and that her safety, welfare and comfort is your greatest joy to provide.

This attitude is as relevant for female therapists as to male ones and I hope that, with this commitment to feminism advancing healthy masculinity, the Core Conditions and the lover's mentality, all massage therapists will be able to successfully create a thriving massage therapy practice in the service of womankind.

CHAPTER THREE

Open Your Mind

Moving on from what was mentioned in the previous chapter regarding the "lover's mentality", it is also helpful for therapists to be a lot more open-minded on what client behaviour they will allow in the massage room.

This is not an excuse for a laissez-faire attitude towards ethics. There is a tightrope that the therapist must walk. Too much "professional facade", by-the-book-no-matter-what attitude and uncomfortable body language and hesitation by the therapist will do little to ease the female client, who may well be a trauma survivor. She has experienced a lifetime under the patriarchy and misogyny of clueless men and expects her therapist to be different.

On the other hand, too free and easy an attitude, with hands everywhere in some well-meant but misguided attempt to "heal" her of her trauma by giving her a happy ending is just asking for trouble. You might as well hang a sign around your neck saying, "SUE ME NOW!"

So where's the happy medium? FOLLOW HER LEAD.

Remember, #MeToo teaches us that it is not the absence or presence of sexuality that determines whether an experience is good or bad, at least in the eyes of women. It is the absence or presence of HER CONTROL. You must, absolutely, at all costs, establish her control over what happens in the massage room. Just doing this will drastically reduce your chances of getting sued. Once her control has been established, THERE IS NO WOMAN stupid enough to be allowed to dictate everything and then later complain about it. In fact, I have been shocked and dismayed by the sheer number of women who have reported that this was the first time she's ever been allowed to decide anything regarding her body, sexually or

14

otherwise; women, who may, in one massage session, tell you that she's had seven boyfriends, then in the next session, say, "Oh, my goodness, this is the first time I've felt this", that makes you think, so what did the seven boyfriends do? Plus, I'm not talking about "this" being some sexual thing – it could be a perfectly innocuous, normal massage stroke that you would do to anybody or even just your mental attention to her body during your work. It could very well be the first time anyone's bothered to give loving attention to the side of her leg or the first time anyone's asked her whether she wants a faster or slower stroke. I have been appalled and heartbroken at the number of women who slog on through life carrying the most dreadful shame about their bodies, even women who, outwardly, appear to be reasonably attractive, successful women in other areas of their life.

I want you to be shocked and appalled with me; to be absolutely aghast at this. This is dreadful. So establishing her control over what happens is absolutely essential. You should regard failure to do so as absolute death to your practice; without it, your attempts at massaging, healing, improving her life are a waste of time – you'll be "just like all the rest" in her eyes. Look at her control over the experience with shock and awe, as though it were the lifeblood of your approach – without it, you will die. It's that important.

That given, then what? You will need to be extremely attentive to your own behaviour and to hers. Women, in general, are more sensitive to their surroundings and the "whole picture" of the environment they are in – sights, sounds, smells, feelings. Men tend to be "zero in" types who narrowly focus on one sensation at a time.

All therapists, male or female, should therefore learn to both monitor how their own behaviour is upholding or limiting client control over the session and also be able to pay attention at the same time to body language clues emanating from the client, such as expressions of comfort vs discomfort, surrender and relaxation vs resistance and tenseness, on an ongoing basis as the session progresses.

To this end, I recommend that all therapists wanting to specialize in women's massage should learn MINDFULNESS.

Mindfulness is a meditative practice with roots in yogic tradition that has been used as a form of stress relief for many years. That, in itself, is useful for massage, since most massages purport to be de-stressing and relaxing to experience. However, that is the client's benefit. Ours is the practice of being attentive to the sights and sounds around us. Usually, in mindfulness, this is done by focusing on one's own breathing. We should do this in the massage room. Alternatively, you can focus on the client's breathing in order to maintain your own focus on her. You can also ask the client to practice mindfulness, either during the initial interview before a massage session or at the beginning of the session, by telling her to focus on her own breathing and the sensations of the massage. If her mind wanders off, she can then return to focus on her breathing. With both you and the client doing this, amazing results can happen. I will go into this in more detail in the next chapter.

With all this in place, I can now recommend that, at this point, you should indeed learn to be more open-minded at the breadth of female sexual expression. This can be achieved by learning about the stages of female sexual arousal and the psychology of female sexual attraction, such as issues like masculine-feminine polarity, mind-body connection, the menstrual cycle and ovulation, hormone fluctuations, age differences and the like.

This is NOT to offer her "optional extras" to your advertised service. Rather, it is so that you become more familiar and comfortable with what these expressions look, sound and feel like, so that, if and when they happen, you don't feel uncomfortable, awkward, scared, angry, hurt or otherwise experience any negative emotion that will transmit through your hands to her and thereby ruin her massage experience.

Women have had enough of men dictating their sexuality or being awkward when it is shown. You must be DIFFERENT. You must be CONFIDENT. So get used to it.

MASSAGING WOMEN

You might think that this advice runs counter to the message of #MeToo – that, now that the truth is out, we all need to be more wary, be more careful, less sexuality should be permitted, we need to double down to avoid harassment, and...

STOP, STOP! TURN BACK! You're going the wrong way!

That's NOT the message of #MeToo, so stop thinking it is. If that's still your attitude, then you're still numbered among the clueless dweebs who "just don't get it". #MeToo is about women's EMPOWERMENT and CONTROL OF THE NARRATIVE that says that men know best about what women should do with their bodies or how, when or where that body should express itself. If you attempt to back out and away from massaging women, then you walk away from a sexual harassment claim and walk straight into a sex discrimination claim. The only way out is through – not up, down or around. Stop avoiding the issue!

It's far better for you to get familiar with the idea that, when you give women control of the massage experience, there is likely to often be a sexual element to her resulting physical expression. Get comfortable with this possibility. Indeed, the more comfortable you are with it, the more it will happen. It's a positive feedback cycle.

Further, when she sees you are not fazed by this but instead, hold space for her to do so, then she feels a transforming relief that is palpable. You, too, will also benefit. When you see her relief, you will feel reassured that all is well. You can then proceed with the massage in confidence. The cycle will then begin again. As these cycles repeat, a greater vulnerability will take hold. You, whether male or female, can then channel this vulnerability into increased mindfulness and focusing more deeply on the Core Conditions and thus both you and her enter into an upward spiral of greater and greater healing. It's absolutely awesome and not just for her. You, too, will be transformed and will come away from the experience amazed by your healing ability and absolutely exhilarated at your ability to heal women.

So don't be afraid to learn about female sexuality – it's powerful but it

17

never killed anyone; and it won't kill you or your practice, for that matter, if you treat it with the respect it deserves.

Women vary greatly in their response. Some women won't want anything sexual to happen at all and feel safest without it – way too triggering. Others will be overtly sexual, brusque and rude about it even, testing you to see how far they can go before you start feeling uncomfortable, then sneering at your perceived failure if you hesitate. Most clients will fall somewhere in the middle of this range. Do you think you can handle it?

What if I'm not sure if what she's doing is sexual or not? LEARN FEMALE SEXUALITY!
How should I start? LOVER'S MENTALITY!
How will I know what's happening with her? MINDFULNESS!
How will I know if I'm doing all right? FOLLOW HER LEAD!
What if I find it hard to agree with her behaviour? CORE CONDITIONS!

Where's your Unconditional Positive Regard?

So this is the bulk of the work of massaging women in the massage room – maintaining this delicate balance. However, if you cultivate an open mindedness towards all this, it will be a lot easier and, even if you sometimes fall, you will fall forward, not back.

CHAPTER FOUR

Massage Her Mindfully

So now we turn our attention somewhat away from you and onto her. WE have established the approach and attitude and mentality YOU should have in this work before you even start; now let's move into the massage room and get started.

In the last chapter, there was a brief introduction to mindfulness and here it is again – it is a meditative technique where we listen, see and use our five senses to truly take in and appreciate what is going on around us, in order to be rooted in the present, rather than have our minds wandering off into the past or the future. ETERNITY IS NOW.

The usual method is to sit upright in a chair or to lie down or whatever is comfortable for you and to tune into the sound of your own breathing. Then you pay attention to sights, sounds, smells, tastes, touches going on around you. You keep this up for half an hour a day as a formal practice. Whenever your mind wanders, bring it back to the breath. There's no need to hurry, get angry or impatient with it and there should be a mild curiosity at what it is your mind wanders off to, not judging or assessing it but letting it just glide right by before returning to the breath. Practitioners use a range of meditations – a Body Scan means to sense feeling in every part of your body, starting with your right big toe, then left, then all toes, then various places on the foot, before moving up the body to cover everything. You can use a Raisin Meditation, spending a long time examining the tastes, textures and feels of a raisin as you eat it and reflecting on all the stages of producing the raisin, from growing it as a grape on a vine somewhere, to a farmer plucking it, drying it out, then it getting shipped and packed into boxes, distributed to the supermarket where you bought it and you buying it. You can try Meditative Yoga, as well as other meditations you can do if you experience adverse or strong reactions to mindfulness.

19

One particular type of mindfulness meditation relevant to massage therapy is one where it is possible to reduce mental or physical pain or stress, where we are encouraged to "lean into" the pain rather than avoid it. One can also develop an informal practice in day-to-day life of practising being mindful while walking along the street, eating a meal or other daily life events.

I advocate that you get into this to add to your women's massage practice. You can also recommend that your client take up the practice, too, since the science of de-stressing that is behind mindfulness is considerable.

However, the main thrust I want to get into is that which I mentioned in the last chapter, where you use your mindfulness in your massage session as a way to be able to be simultaneously present to your own behaviour and in tune with hers without having to constantly switch your mental attention back and forth manually between the two to maintain the balance between ethics and client control described in that chapter. This ease and fluidity takes some time to develop and to achieve it will mean that you must take up mindfulness as a habit yourself.

Begin by first using mindfulness to assess the room before the session starts – is it too hot or too cold? Are there distracting noises? Is the breeze from a fan likely to assist or irritate the client? Is the lighting too bright and clinical – should it perhaps be dimmed to create a more intimate or private atmosphere? Are there any unpleasant fast food smells arising from a canteen or local restaurant coming in through the window? What about tastes – have you brushed your teeth since lunch? Touches – are your fingertips unnecessarily rough or calloused? Hang nails – file them down!

Much of this comes under general good practice anyway but get into the habit of using mindfulness for it for your own benefit, just to get you started on being mindful before the client walks in the door.

Once the client has arrived and the massage has begun, you will need to constantly monitor three things – the massage strokes themselves, your demeanour and her reactions. At first, using mindfulness to scroll your
20

brain through Core Conditions, Lover's Mentality, Follow Her Lead and Female Sexuality, then check in on her, then manage the strokes, then back through those four things again and keep doing this around and around for an hour's session will be mentally tiring. However, make the effort! It won't be long before your brain starts using shortcuts, like mental images, rather than the actual words I wrote in this Guide, to help you and then these will be parsed down further to just "feelings" for each one where you just sense that things are OK or not and you're able to react much more rapidly and fluidly to things as they arise, rather than mentally going through a list of checkboxes. You'll be able to react to anything adverse lightning fast without losing focus on what's important by doing so – and the client should be satisfied.

There's much more to this than meets the eye but that's enough to get you started for now and, by doing this, you will rapidly escalate your in-session awareness to that of most women, which will, in turn, align the massage experience you offer her to one much closer to the reality of the female experience of life.

A Quick-Start Guide for Therapists in the Age of #MeToo

CHAPTER FIVE

Follow Her Lead

As mentioned before, this is the most important part as far as your client is concerned. Everything before is just preparation, leading up to this; preparing you, so you are ready for this moment. So let's start.

I am assuming that you have done the intake interview to assess the client's health and any specific presenting concerns and complaints, that all paperwork has been filed upfront and all necessary procedures done, so that now we are at the point where the client just walks through the door and we start.

Begin by NOT telling the client to remove clothes. This is the most important first step – never skip it. It is the foundation of this whole approach. Instead, invite the client to sit on the massage chair or lie down on the table with all the clothes they walk in with, including any outer garments for the weather – everything.

Start the massage. Typically, this means knead the shoulders if the client is seated or start working her back if she is lying down. Usually, if she is wearing any clothes for the weather, she will immediately volunteer to take them off. Let her do so. Resume the massage.

Assuming she is lying face down, continue massaging through her blouse or top. Some minutes usually pass before she offers to remove this also. During this time, she is assessing the safety situation, your demeanor and

22

the environment. Once she is satisfied with this assessment, her offer will then come. Say, "You can if you want to but you don't have to if you don't want to". Let her decide. Presuming your demeanor is unchanged and remains friendly, she will eventually do so.

Repeat this procedure for all outer clothing until she is in the normal state of undress required of a regular massage session. You will have to massage those body parts through the clothing before she offers to take them off. DO NOT race through massaging different body parts for a few minutes at a time, to get the required amount of clothes off, just to get her to this point. This point is NOT important. Typically, the more she takes off, the longer time she will take in deciding about each article of clothing and in assessing safety levels.

In a normal massage session, you would start by simply saying, "Please take off your shirt, lie down on the table", similar to a doctor, then go straight to draping. That approach indicates that you're the boss and that you will be the one deciding when things happen, in what order, plus there's a tendency to think, "ethics = draping". In the light of #MeToo and the assumption that every woman is a trauma survivor of such horrendous things as assault and rape, such an approach looks laughably inadequate for most women. Where's her control or input?

So abandon the idea of "having to get her into a state of undress, then drape her up, then start". Once she has removed enough clothes to allow skin-to-skin contact, get started with the oil. Don't worry that her lower body is still fully clothed. Massage the parts she has agreed to expose.

Assuming you have started with her back, the next issue will be the bra strap. It's in the way. Act like this is totally fine, jumping your fingers over it to avoid getting oil on it and just carry on in your merry way. DO NOT get huffy and puffy or act like it's this huge inconvenience or start sighing

A Quick-Start Guide for Therapists in the Age of #MeToo

or, even worse, attempt to rub and stroke under it or any of that rubbish. You're telegraphing what you want her to do. Ahem! You're directing the speed and the action, aren't you? In this approach, SHE'S the boss. She decides this junk. She decides the action and the speed at which it happens. Understand that a bra is an item of underwear designed to cover up her secondary sexual organs. While those organs are underneath her in a face-down position, that's still a major deal for a woman, especially one who may have been abused. Back off! Everything she decides is fine with you. The customer is always right. Where's your empathy?

Typically, she'll take her time deciding whether to unhook the bra strap or not for you. However, assuming you haven't blown it via the abovementioned attitude problem, practicality will win out and she'll lay the bra straps so that the bra is in place but the straps are lying each side of her on the table. Resume the massage.

Now, if you experience a situation where a woman adamantly refuses to undo it, this is usually your fault for not establishing Core Conditions or else not paying attention somehow via Mindfulness. Re-establish this at once and continue massaging with the bra strap in place until she feels able to trust you enough that she takes it off.

Also, do not help her to undo the clip. Let her do the whole action. It allows her greater ownership of her own behaviour, which increases her confidence in herself and in you.

Don't be in a hurry to move things along. She's not stupid – she knows she paid for an hour's massage to achieve a certain outcome, whether that be general relaxation, knot release or whatever the presenting problem is. If she knows the time is limited, she will pace things so as to achieve what she wants in the time available, subject to what you told her in the intake interview. If she paid for an hour's full-body massage, she's not going to

24

spend 45 minutes hesitating to undo her bra. On the other hand, if she complains of a knot in her calf muscle, she'll be questioning why you think the bra strap is so important. Trust in her judgement.

Once you have completed massaging one area of exposed skin, you may now drape it before moving onto the next clothed area and repeating this whole process.

Continue this process until the massage is complete.

A Quick-Start Guide for Therapists in the Age of #MeToo

CHAPTER SIX

Awaken Her Healing

The process described in the last chapter is the main, basic, practical approach of this Quick-Start Guide. It is appropriate for a first session and all subsequent ones with the same client.

However, it must be said that this whole process of Mindfulness in massage, Core Conditions of empathy, genuineness and unconditional positive regard, Lover's Mentality towards women and Follow Her Lead can often create a "wow" factor in women at your skills and abilities. This, in turn, will usually lead to her telling all her friends, creating for you an ample supply of new clientele. If you work in a clinic, there will be demand from clients to get you as their therapist and not one of the others. If you are in private practice, then you'll suddenly find yourself with a busy schedule of house calls.

However, consonant with this will be a tendency for the client to go one step further – some women in every session, others just occasionally. Each time the client arrives, she will have that much more trust in you – her ability to trust the process will be stronger, her comfort more established. So this will create an expectation that she can relax more, cover issues she didn't the first time, go over old health problems that may resurface and other physiologically related matters.

Further, she will likely discuss with you more intimate details of her life, talking about ex-boyfriends, what they did together, dates that went badly, guys she met, etc. It's important as a therapist for you to let her do all this without feeling uncomfortable. This is where your knowledge of Female Sexuality becomes relevant.

Ultimately, on a larger scale, what is happening here is that you are being included as a member of the sisterhood, the whisper network of women around the world that keeps them safe from dangerous, patriarchal, misogynistic men. If you're a female therapist, well, you're already included but if you are a man, then being included should be regarded as a seriously major, huge deal. You will be expected to maintain absolute secrecy and remain absolutely faithful to her safety, since some women who are still in abusive relationships when you meet them as clients will need it as a matter of life and death. You don't know the full ins and outs of her situation and many women keep even other women on only a "need-to-know" basis. You do not repeat what you hear to anyone.

Absolutely the worst thing you can do is to act like her conversation during the massage session is some kind of distraction to your work. Ahem! Are you not a healer? Women express themselves emotionally and that, in itself, is a form of healing. We're here to serve. Let her speak. Don't act like you're just this "professional" - you are but remember the Core Conditions – where's your genuineness?

Now, finally, no Quick-Start Guide to massaging women would be complete without covering the situation where all this personal disclosure, following her lead, letting her decide how far to go and all the other aspects of this approach we have covered leads to a situation where the woman expresses herself in sexual ways in the massage room. What's recommended here?

Your basic approach to this issue should be this – you, yourself, as either a male or female therapist, will never do anything sexual to the client in the

27

massage room as a paid service. Absolutely nothing. You must pay no attention to all such requests for the duration of the session. If she insists, refuse.

That said, you need to be open-minded to the possibility that all this control that you have given her and the various features of this approach may well lead to her becoming increasingly confident that she can explore sexual avenues of relief in front of you by herself while you continue a normal massage service.

Typically, this will tend to manifest when you turn her over so she is facing up and, with her breasts and groin area suitably draped and you continuing to massage normally, she decides by herself to start touching her breasts under the drape with her hands. Depending on their levels of comfort, other women may arch their back, start touching between their legs under the drape or even full-on start stimulating themselves. There could be vocalisation or deeper breathing.

Ignore all this and continue massaging normally. Make no changes, body language communication or indication that anything out of the ordinary is happening.

The features of the approach outlined in this Guide are, in many ways, a method of massage therapy that gives power to women to control what happens in the massage room. You need to realise that, ultimately, in this life, that outside the massage room, women are constantly being controlled and the number one reason is because of their sexuality. So be philosophical about the fact that she's not trying to make you feel awkward but that all giving of power to women in a theatre where physical touch is involved is likely to end up this way eventually. You can't expect to give more and more power to women while touching them and vainly imagine that somehow this isn't going end up with her doing a

28

bit of exploration at some point. Use your Lover's Mentality and knowledge of Female Sexuality to help you to realise that this is an amazing thing for her, that you have achieved this level of comfort for her, that you have held space for her, created an environment of safety for her and now she wants to play. Understand that being with women is one of the greatest pleasures of life and watching her orgasm is your reward for your dedicated service in creating this opportunity for her. Remember, you have given her control – let her use it. For sure, she won't sue you!

A Quick-Start Guide for Therapists in the Age of #MeToo

Conclusion

So there you have it! My approach for massaging women, all broken-down into a bitesize little Quick-Start Guide that you can use to transform your female clients' lives and bring them the healing that they have always wanted!

I invite you to subscribe to my e-mail newsletter (if you have not done so already) and check out my YouTube videos and blog website! The blog and YouTube channel are at -

Thanks for reading and have a great life! Wishing you all the best for the future, I remain,

yours faithfully,

Oliver Chapman, DipCPC, CPT
Certified Life Coach

MASSAGING WOMEN

About the Author

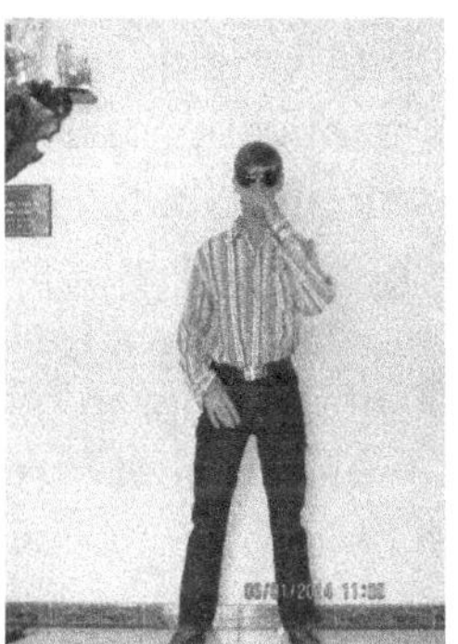

Oliver Chapman is a 46-year-old British massage therapist, blogger, YouTuber, Certified Life Coach, Personal Trainer, personal development expert Good Men Project Weekly Columnist and teacher based in Ho Chi Minh City, Vietnam. He is married to a Vietnamese wife and has one son.

His love for his teenage students and his desire to help them live a better life inspired him to move into writing. He has now expanded this mission to include feminism and LGBT rights, as many of the issues raised by these topic impact his students and others he wishes to help.

This is his eighth book. His dream is to use the money he gains from the sale of this book to improve the lives of his students, women and LGBT people. His plan is to set up a drop-in centre to inspire them to become the people they have always wanted to be and to give them the dream life they have always desired!

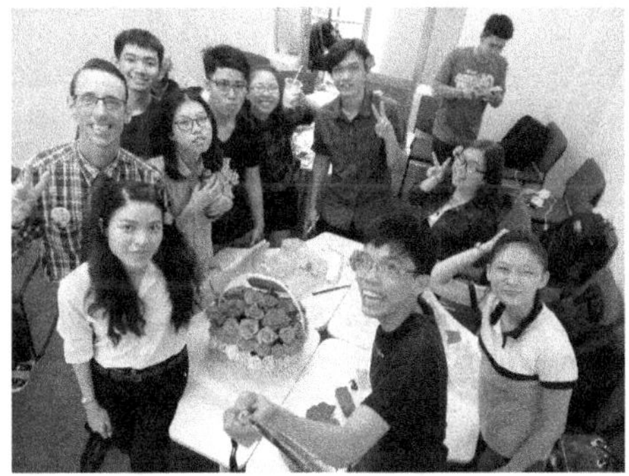

A Quick-Start Guide for Therapists in the Age of #MeToo

MASSAGING WOMEN

Ebook disclaimer

by SEQ Legal

(1) Introduction
This disclaimer governs the use of this ebook. By using this ebook, you accept this disclaimer in full.

(2) Credit
This disclaimer was created using an SEQ Legal template.

(3) No advice
The ebook contains advice on massage therapy. The information is not professional advice, and should not be treated as such. You must not rely on the information in the ebook as an alternative to advice on massage therapy matters from an appropriately qualified professional. If you have any specific questions about any massage therapy matter you should consult an appropriately qualified professional.

A Quick-Start Guide for Therapists in the Age of #MeToo

(4) No representations or warranties
To the maximum extent permitted by applicable law and subject to section
6 below, we exclude all representations, warranties, undertakings and
guarantees relating to the ebook.
Without prejudice to the generality of the foregoing paragraph, we do not
represent, warrant, undertake or guarantee: that the information in
the ebook is correct, accurate, complete or non-misleading; that the use of
the guidance in the ebook will lead to any particular outcome or result;
or in particular, that by using the guidance in the ebook you will achieve a
better life for yourself or any other person you may share it with.

(5) Limitations and exclusions of liability
The limitations and exclusions of liability set out in this section and
elsewhere in this disclaimer: are subject to section 6 below; and govern all
liabilities arising under the disclaimer or in relation to the ebook, including
liabilities arising in contract, in tort (including negligence) and for breach
of statutory duty.
We will not be liable to you in respect of any losses arising out of any
event or events beyond our reasonable control.
We will not be liable to you in respect of any business losses, including
without limitation loss of or damage to profits, income, revenue, use,
production, anticipated savings, business, contracts, commercial
opportunities or goodwill.
We will not be liable to you in respect of any loss or corruption of any
data, database or software.
We will not be liable to you in respect of any special, indirect or
consequential loss or damage.

(6) Exceptions
Nothing in this disclaimer shall: limit or exclude our liability for death or
personal injury resulting from negligence; limit or exclude our liability for
fraud or fraudulent misrepresentation; limit any of our liabilities in any
way that is not permitted under applicable law; or exclude any of our
liabilities that may not be excluded under applicable law.

A Quick-Start Guide for Therapists in the Age of #MeToo

(7) Severability
If a section of this disclaimer is determined by any court or other competent authority to be unlawful and/or unenforceable, the other sections of this disclaimer continue in effect.
If any unlawful and/or unenforceable section would be lawful or enforceable if part of it were deleted, that part will be deemed to be deleted, and the rest of the section will continue in effect.

(8) Law and jurisdiction
This disclaimer will be governed by and construed in accordance with Vietnamese law, and any disputes relating to this disclaimer will be subject to the exclusive jurisdiction of the courts of the Socialist Republic of Vietnam.

(9) Our details
In this disclaimer, "we" means (and "us" and "our" refer to) Oliver Chapman of Flat 410, Lo A1, C/C A3, Phan Xich Long Street, Ward
7, Phu Nhuan District, Ho Chi Minh City, Socialist Republic of Vietnam.

A Quick-Start Guide for Therapists in the Age of #MeToo